Beyond the Mailbox

Beyond the Mailbox

A Life with Chronic Illness

PAT GAVULA

For Pat Soychak who said,

"You have to get this information out there".

Table of Contents

He had to give up work and embrace the sorry occupation known as taking care of one's self. At first he was greatly disgusted; it appeared to him that it was not himself in the least that he was taking care of, but an uninteresting and uninterested person with whom he had nothing in common. This person, however, improved on acquaintance, and Ralph grew at least to have a certain grudging tolerance, and even undemonstrative respect, for him. Misfortune makes strange bedfellows, and our young man, feeling that he had something at stake in the matter – it usually seemed to him to be his reputation for common sense – devoted to his unattractive protégé an amount of attention of which note was duly taken, and which had at least the effect of keeping the poor fellow alive.

Henry James *The Portrait of a Lady*

Too tired for company,
You seek a solitude
You are too tired to fill.

Dag Hammerskjold *Markings*

Introduction

This is a book about my experience living with Myalgic Encephalomyelitis (ME), commonly known as Chronic Fatigue Syndrome (CFS).

The intent of this book is to give hope to my fellow travelers on the ME road, to give travelers on other roads some insight into the ME journey and how they might read the map by which those with ME guide their lives, and to portray the physical, emotional, spiritual, and social struggles of living with chronic illness.

I write from the perspective of someone who has lived the greater part of my adult life with ME to one extent or another. I also write as a former physician assistant. From that perspective I can speak with a modicum of expertise in medical matters and about the medical world. I also write from the other side of the stethoscope in my role as a patient. A Master's degree in theology and training in spiritual direction help me write from theological and spiritual perspectives.

I hope that all these aspects of myself blend together in this writing and pull together various themes related to living with chronic illness in general and ME in particular.

This is not a medical book nor will it give you the magic you need to return your life to normal should you be living with ME. It is not intended as a substitute for seeking qualified medical consultation for whatever symptoms you may be experiencing. I do hope, however, that it gives you some reason to get up again tomorrow.

This is my story. Yours is different. Honor mine and honor yours.

A Bit About Me

From my perspective there are two kinds of people in the world: those who awaken and say, "Good Morning, God!", and those who awaken and say, "Good god. Morning." I belong to the latter group.

Facing another day is difficult when it is likely to be just like the previous innumerable of days of low energy, poor stamina, and the struggle to accomplish life's tasks. Can I stand long enough to brush my teeth? Do I even bother flossing today, or only if I sit down to do it?

Day after relentless day of this prompts one to think about the purpose of one's life. What value is there to a life that is primarily focused on slogging from one task to another with no light at the end of the tunnel? It gives a new twist to the term "tunnel vision".

For those living with a chronic illness the world becomes very small. Our energy is so focused on getting life's basics completed – washing up, doing the daily dental routine, perhaps changing out of pjs, getting something to eat – that little is left for anything or anyone else.

As of this writing I am 68 years old and have lived with ME for 35 years. I used to be well. I used to be slim and trim. For several years I was a runner. After my running days were over I would instead go for a brisk three mile walk with my dog, do chores around the house, leave early for work, go to the pool and swim

¾ of a mile, and then pound the floors of the emergency room for my shift as a physician assistant. Go hiking for the day? No problem. Stuff a backpack with some food and go cross-country skiing for the day? No problem.

Then I started to experience knee pain. First it was just after mowing the lawn. Then it was present regardless of activity or rest. Then, when I was swimming, I'd feel as if I was tethered to the opposite end of the pool or that I was swimming through gelatin. I'd get out of the pool and almost crawl over to a chair to sit and rest for a few minutes until I had the strength to walk to the locker room. What was happening to my body? I'd have episodes where I was exhausted, had muscle aches, joint pain, and chills. Then I'd be right back to normal. Back to walking, and hiking, and swimming without a care in the world. I was fine. Then I wasn't and I haven't been since.

At a point early in my illness I had some sort of viral episode. I awoke with a mild sore throat. If memory serves, it was a Friday and I had a potluck planned for Sunday. I had just put the invitation out there, no RSVP required. We'd do with whatever and whoever showed up. As I was out shopping for food I started to feel much worse. I wasn't sure I'd make it out of the store but I did, rested in the car for a few minutes and then drove home and called my doctor. She saw me that afternoon, did a rapid Strep test, which was negative, and drew blood for a CBC (complete blood count). I remember that it was winter because it was unusual for me to be sitting in the living room taking off layer after layer of clothes and then later putting them all back on. I suppose I had had a fever which then resolved in response to some Tylenol or Advil I had taken.

The next day my doctor called to ask how I was feeling and suggested I cancel the potluck since I had a white blood cell count of over 38,000. (Normal range is 5,000 to 10,000/ml depending on various factors.) I was tired but no longer feeling acutely ill and went ahead with my plans. Afterwards, although my blood tests returned to baseline and I'd occasionally have some "normal" days, they started to become fewer and farther apart.

I often wonder about the role of stress in not only the onset of my symptoms but in their continuation and exacerbation. I don't think it was a coincidence that my symptoms started when I was suddenly responsible for the upkeep and management of the first house I owned alone. It was spring when my symptoms started. The lawn was growing, and the mower broke. Well, actually the power cord was chewed by my darling puppy dog, Josie, in her hours of boredom while I was at work. The lawn was rapidly getting out of control and mower repair people were backed up with work. So, when the mower finally did get fixed I had a tall lawn to mow which put stress on body and spirit.

Work was not going well and I was to lose that job in the fall of that year and then start working in the emergency room, a position for which I felt totally inadequate and unprepared. Life seemed to move from stressor to stressor. Is it unreasonable to think that my body wouldn't react in some negative way? I feel very strongly that whatever is wrong with my body today is simply the result of what it has been through over the past 35 years. I feel it is damaged beyond repair.

Over the years I've consulted with doctors in many specialties and have tried many conventional and non-traditional remedies but to no avail. My symptoms have, however, continued to interfere with my ability to work and to live a full life. Over time I was forced to give up all the physical activities I enjoyed. My world slowly became smaller and smaller, confined closer and closer to the house side of the mailbox and less and less frequently beyond. All of my limited energy went into simply surviving.

The cognitive deficits are the most difficult to endure. Memory loss, no longer absorbing music like a sponge, word searching (and not finding), computing difficulties (I did learn multiplication tables once, didn't I?), loss of spatial relationships, slow processing – this is the mind of a much older person but I was still young and experiencing these deficits starting in my 30s. How was this also my mind? How could I present myself as competent when I no longer felt that way?

I wonder if it is more challenging for a woman, and a single woman in particular, living alone, to live with chronic health problems. It is well known that women are not taken as seriously as men when presenting to health care providers with symptoms. And if those symptoms are mysterious and defy diagnosis it is easier to attribute them to being "all in your head" or to cure "if you'd just get a life" if the one presenting is a woman.

I may never know what caused the onset of my symptoms or their continuation. I do know that I was constantly faced with what seemed an impossible choice: take care of myself or pay the bills. Paying the bills won.

This is how ME is manifested in me:

- Unrelenting fatigue that sometimes makes it difficult to do even the simplest of tasks
- A sense of total exhaustion: mental, physical, emotional, spiritual
- Postural intolerance. Sometimes I can't tolerate sitting or standing for more than a minute
- Non-restorative sleep: I never, ever, ever feel as if I have slept or slept enough regardless of how long I have slept
- Chills, even if it's 90 degrees outside
- Cognitive issues: memory deficits – putting information in my memory and retrieving information from my memory; word recall, difficulties with calculation. Sometimes I'm not able to read a novel or work on a crossword puzzle.

- Noise sensitivity and intolerance of crowds or even being in the company of more than two other people
- Day/night reversal
- Loss of appetite and limited food intake, yet I'm obese
- Exercise intolerance
- Over-reaction to activity or stressors of any kind (good or bad) which can send me to bed for days
- An overall sense of weakness
- Muscle aches and joint pain

It's not a pretty picture but it is my reality.

ME is now, finally, recognized by the CDC and by the Social Security Administration as a legitimate illness. It has the all-important diagnosis code that makes it real. Prior to that recognition it was quite difficult for people with ME to be awarded disability benefits. I'm sure my age and the length of my symptomatology helped my cause back in 2013 when I finally had to stop working. I was fortunate enough to be awarded disability benefits on my first attempt. Although I wish I were able to be gainfully employed I am, nonetheless, grateful for the Social Security benefits that allow me to maintain my independence.

So, What Is Myalgic Encephalomyelitis?

Myalgic Encephalomyelitis (ME) is a chronic illness of unknown origin. There is no specific diagnostic test for ME. It is a "diagnosis of exclusion" meaning that after all the tests have been done and no cause has been found for one's symptoms, the person may be diagnosed with ME.

The Centers for Disease Control and Prevention (CDC) describes ME as "a disabling and complex illness". It is an illness that disrupts every aspect of one's life. At times it can prevent a person from earning a living or even from sitting up in bed or being able to feed themselves. No one has yet discovered what causes ME and it has no known cure.

The primary symptom is profound fatigue that is not relieved by rest or any amount of sleep. It is fatigue that NEVER goes away. It is there from the moment of awakening to the moment of falling asleep. It is there through every meal and every errand. It is there through every conversation and every quiet moment. It is there through every attempt to read a book and through every decision of what to wear.

People with ME frequently experience post-exertional malaise (PEM). In other words, if they exert themselves too much, they pay for it. And just what is "too much"? It may be something as simple as taking a shower, or picking up a few groceries, or putting new linens on the bed, or chatting on the phone. Activities that would never have been a problem in the past can now potentially send the person with ME to bed for days or weeks or months. This is often referred to as "crashing". And it feels that way. It feels like running into a brick wall or being hit with the worst flu of one's life. People with ME may be profoundly exhausted even by the thought of turning over in bed. They may have no appetite. They may not be able read or perhaps even listen to the radio or hold a conversation. Add on top of that chills and body aches, and perhaps a low-grade fever. With the flu or a bad cold a person can be fairly certain that the worst symptoms will abate in a few days, but a crash can last for a long time and perhaps never end.

Many people with ME have sleep issues. They may have difficulty falling asleep or staying asleep. Their sleep is "non-restorative", meaning that they never feel refreshed or restored, even after a full night's sleep. Some experience "day/night reversal", meaning that they tend to fall asleep late and sleep late. They're like night shift workers in that they fall asleep as the sun is rising and awaken around noon or early afternoon. This presents real difficulties for those trying to work a day job, if they can work at all.

Another prominent feature of ME is what is commonly referred to as "brain fog". A person experiencing "brain fog" has difficulty thinking clearly, recalling words or names, placing information in the memory or retrieving information from it, making decisions, figuring things out, reading a novel or a newspaper, solving a puzzle, engaging in a conversation, thinking on their feet.

In addition, many people with ME experience orthostatic intolerance, sometimes referred to as "postural orthostatic tachycardic syndrome" or POTS. People with POTS get dizzy with standing or even sitting. They may feel lightheaded or weak or feel an urgent need to sit down or lie down.

Other symptoms may include sore throat, headaches, muscle aches or muscle weakness, joint pain, shortness of breath, heart problems, digestive issues, and new sensitivities to food or to odors, light, or noise.

In sum, ME is a total body illness.

What's It Like?

Living with Myalgic Encephalomyelitis is like riding a roller coaster blindfolded. One has no idea if the symptoms are going up or down, how soon, how quickly, if/when they will even off, or if the ride will ever end.

Living with ME is like living with a body that is not running on all cylinders, like the power has gone out, accompanied by the daily or perhaps hourly decision of how to spend a thimbleful of energy. One's world becomes very, very small and there is the risk of it becoming so insular that the outside world becomes a foreign place, a frightening and unknown place full of people who don't or can't understand why the ill person is not able to participate in the same way they are able.

It is a life of going through the motions, and the emotions.

It is a jigsaw puzzle with pieces missing.

It is being caught in a spiral or cycle of grief from season to season and year to year.

It is like living in a perpetual Lent – a dying, a deprivation, a sacrificing, a transformation, a dark journey into the depths.

It's like having an errant thread weaving through the otherwise beautiful tapestry of your life.

It is like walking on a narrow balance beam where it takes very little to teeter on the brink of falling – falling apart, falling into depression, falling into debt, falling into homelessness, falling into despair — because not falling — keeping balance — takes energy, energy that is in poor supply.

I wrote this simple comparison one day:

Well Person:	**Me:**
I'm off to work again.	I'm off to bed again.
I'm going shopping.	I'm going to rest.
It's payday.	It's disability check day.
Ugh! Three loads of laundry.	My only laundry is pajamas.
I got so much done today!	I sat up for ten minutes today.
What do you want for dinner?	Don't even mention food.
...and then she said....	Frankly, my dear....
Phew! It's hot today.	Why do I have chills?
Remember when....	No, I don't.
It's hard living with a person who's sick.	It's hard living with a person who is well.
I got caught in the rain. I'm soaked.	When was the last time I could stand long enough to take a shower?

଼

Chronic illness changes one's self-image: from being competent and able to being incompetent and unable; from being one who can to one who can't; from someone with hopes and dreams to someone whose only hope and dream is to die as soon as possible since this is the only relief from this life of chronic disease.

Those with chronic illness live a life of continually grieving lost abilities. That list, for me, includes the loss of the ability to tolerate physical activities such as hiking, biking, walking any significant distance, traveling very far (even as a passenger), swimming; the loss of the ability to stand for any significant period of time, sometimes even enough time for a shower or be in line at the grocery store; the loss of the ability to lead the singing in church or participate in the community chorus; the loss of the ability to plan for tomorrow, loss of confidence in my body and of good body image, loss of a job, loss of hobbies that require sitting or standing for periods of time, and on some days loss of ability to concentrate on reading.

I have experienced the loss of health, of friends and acquaintances, of employment, of income, of the ability to have fun, of the ability to support myself. I have lost brain power, the ability to exercise and thus control my weight, the ability to engage in activities I enjoy. I have lost self-esteem, dreams for the future, the image of myself as useful and intelligent. All these losses cause great sadness and chronic grief or what some refer to as chronic sorrow.

Chronic sorrow is not the same as normal grief nor is it the same as depression. I particularly appreciate Susan Roos's treatment of chronic sorrow in her book of the same name. She writes from her perspective as the mother of children with significant disabilities. Roos describes chronic sorrow as a "living loss". As opposed to the grief one feels after the death of a loved one, the loss of a job, or of one's possessions in a fire, chronic sorrow is the grief one feels for the on-going loss of something that still exists, or someone who is still present, still living. With chronic illness the losses are in one's own being, not external, and therefore unescapable. If one is going to persist in living with a chronic illness one must then also persist in living with the losses associated with that illness. Chronic sorrow means living with chronic sadness.

It can be difficult to tease apart sadness and depression. Although some health care providers have diagnosed me with depression and, at times, I have certainly been clinically depressed and suicidal and have been on anti-depressants, I suspect that the real bases for these experiences were sadness, anger, and fear, especially because I don't feel any differently when I'm not taking anti-depressants. It is not unreasonable for a person to be depressed about living with a chronic illness that has resulted in so many losses which lead to so much grieving. Underneath that depression, or perhaps the cause of that depression and subsequent grieving, are profound sadness, anger, and fear.

Just as there is a fine line between sadness and depression, there is also a fine line between fear and worry. I try to remember the words spoken so often in scripture, "do not be afraid", or "fear not", because except when life and limb are at risk, fear is generally not helpful and can, in fact, be quite destructive.

However, I do worry. I worry about not being able to cope with whatever life throws at me. I don't have much reserve to deal with emergencies or those little (and big) annoyances that happen from time to time like the car unexpectedly ceasing to function or a house issue that needs immediate attention. I don't have the flexibility to respond well to those curve balls that are tossed my way. I almost feel paralyzed when faced with the unexpected.

I worry that I will live a long and boring life. I worry I don't have the resiliency or desire to keep going. I worry that my tendency to withdraw and become a recluse will not be a healthy approach for me. I worry about not having the financial means to support myself until I die.

All these are reasonable fears, I suppose, but become exaggerated for those who are chronically ill and have little reserve.

Returning to the issue of grieving living losses, life with a chronic illness fits in well with Elisabeth Kubler-Ross's stages of death and dying. Setting aside whether these are currently in vogue, they are of some benefit here.

At first, one may deny that health will not return quickly. A person may say, "No way; this is not happening to me". One may withdraw from family and friends overwhelmed by the thought of being so sick. One may even avoid going back to the doctor because if we don't see the doctor then we can pretend the illness does not exist.

Anger may be the next emotion to experience. Illness does not fit with the plan we had for our lives. This is not what one had in mind. It is easy to direct anger in all sorts of directions: family, friends, parents, spouse or partner, our children, our siblings, our doctor, the health care system, our boss, God, and ourselves.

One may be angry because there is no time or money to be sick or because one's plans for the future have been interrupted or dashed forever. We may be angry at ourselves for not seeking a medical opinion earlier or for not heeding the advice of others to do so. Perhaps one has a sense of being punished for past misdeeds or failings – real or imagined. One may be angry at God for allowing such a thing to happen to a good person.

Then one may bargain. One may make promises to oneself, to others, to God in order to get well. One may promise all sorts of things – reasonable and unreasonable – in exchange for wellness.

Depression is often the next step and is a normal response to not getting what one bargained for. One may sulk. One may cry. One may wallow in self-pity. One experiences a sense of great loss when one realizes that health is not just over the horizon. The losses associated with chronic illness are especially cruel because they never go away.

Acceptance is considered the final stage. There's a difference, I feel, between acceptance of a situation and acquiescence to it. In chronic illness, this can be a thin line. I consider acceptance to be an active process and acquiescence to be passive. One acquiesces with an "Oh well, nothing I can do about it" attitude, while one accepts with an "Oh well. OK. I don't like It, but I'll live with it" attitude. I strive for the latter approach.

In sum, living with a chronic illness like ME changes everything about oneself and one's world. It is a life-altering experience.

What Is Wellness?

Compassion is sometimes lacking in the medical profession. I suspect, and I can say this with some credibility having been part of that world for over twenty years, it stems from the fear that, although these professionals are knowledgeable about medical issues, they do not have the power to prevent illness from happening to themselves or their loved ones. This can be terrifying, and that fear can be transferred to patients and colleagues, friends and family. How sad. How sad that it is so easy to forget that we are mortal, that no matter what happens we all die. How sad that some medical professionals consider the death of a patient a personal failure.

How often does a medical professional ask a patient how their blood pressure is, or how their diabetes is, or how their arthritis medication is working but fail to ask the most important question: How are *you*? This was one of my frustrations in working as a physician assistant. My job was to diagnose illness and treat it, not to be interested or concerned about any other aspect of a person's life. Yet no one can bring only part of themselves to the health care provider's office. We are whole beings and need to be treated as such.

For some medical professionals, when a person presents with mysterious symptoms the first inclination is to a diagnosis of mental illness, especially if the patient is a woman. It seems that if the symptoms are not neatly summarized in a medical textbook, don't have a diagnosis code, and don't make sense then the problem itself doesn't exist, or else the person is crazy and the symptoms are all in the person's head. Get a life, we are told. Get into (or out of) a relationship. Take up a hobby. Don't work so hard. Take a vacation. Few practitioners seem to take the approach of "How interesting. How are you coping with this? Let's see if we can figure this out."

People can be demanding of instant diagnosis and instant cure, especially given the money we pay for health insurance and medical care and considering the "advanced" state of medicine in the Western world. Our society wages war on illness – the war on cancer, the war on drugs. What happens when we lose the war? When a person continues to be ill or dies, is that a failure of the health care system or of the patient? There seems to be a need to place blame somewhere. But there is so much more to the human body than we know. We have barely scratched the surface of our understanding of how the body functions and the role of the mind and spirit in wellness and illness.

There certainly is a mental aspect to illness and wellness. The mind is very powerful. Can we will ourselves ill? Can we will ourselves well? Think about the words will and ill, only separated by one letter. And will and well, again only separated by one letter. Are we only one little letter away from illness or wellness? How much power do we have in our minds and spirits to effect healing? And what type of healing? What is healing anyway?

I feel there is a difference between healing and curing. It is not uncommon for these words to be used interchangeably. Many assume that if you are cured you are healed, and vice versa. I would contend that these two conditions can, and often are, very different. A few illnesses and diseases are actually cured. But, primarily, illnesses and diseases are managed with medication or life-style changes or perhaps herbal treatments or another of the non-traditional approaches.

Some may think healing means the illness or condition has gone away. I would call that being cured. Healing is a much more complex process. We can be healed spiritually, emotionally, psychologically, and not at all physically. Many people have been known to utter the, to some, strange thought that "this illness is the best thing that ever happened to me". How can this be? Why would something that sweeps you off your feet (and not in a good way) be a good thing? There must be something to this illness stuff that is beyond the surface, beyond first sight.

I recall having a conversation with an acquaintance who had a condition that, if it progressed, would significantly impair his ability to maintain an independent life. We discussed whether it was right to pray for healing. Such prayers, if not answered as expected, could bring up important theological issues. Are prayers heard? Is there any point to praying? Is there a God, and, if so, is God listening? If I am not healed, does that mean God is punishing me? My friend felt it was probably best to leave healing in the "God realm" and let God decide what kind of healing is best for us. It may be that the healing we need most is not physical. We may be best served by healing relationships or by healing faults within ourselves, rather than having a physical ailment removed and having those other "illnesses" remain. This seems a much more wholistic approach than just praying or hoping or begging that our physical ills disappear.

Having been educated in the medical model in the 1980s and having taught in physician assistant training programs in the 1990s and 2000s I can say with confidence that the psycho-social-spiritual wellbeing of a person was not high on the lists of concerns if it existed as part of the curriculum at all. I hope it is different now. As a patient, I have often found health care providers are more comfortable asking about a patient's sex life than about how their illness affects their day-to-day living, or their self-esteem, or their ability to continue working, or to volunteer at the local thrift shop.

Additionally in my training, there was no course or lecture on death and dying. Our job was to heal, save lives, make things better. The death of a patient was a failure. In a discussion with colleagues about whether or not a medical professional should attend the funeral of a patient the overwhelming opinion was that such an action would be inappropriate. It would reflect poorly on the medical person. It would remind the family of what the medical person was unable to do – save the life of the deceased. It would not bring comfort to the family. It would deflect attention from the grieving survivors to the "incompetent" caregiver. This seems wrong to me. If we accompany a person through their illness, competently and confidently, we should have no qualms about facing the family and, as a fellow mourner, offer condolences and show our respect for the deceased.

As medical advancements have made living to the ripe old age of 90 or 100 not so unusual, we can be deluded into thinking that we will live forever. How shocked we are when someone dies at the age of 66. She was so young, we say, when in the not-so-distant past living to 66 was quite the accomplishment. The medical world is daily expanding its armamentarium of new drugs, new tests, new treatments, such that we wonder if there is any disease that cannot be cured when in reality very few are. Primarily we control disease rather than cure it. So, should death be such a surprise?

I have had the opportunity to lecture to physician assistant (PA) students on how to bring spiritual questions into conversations with patients. My aim was to make them as comfortable asking spiritual questions as they would be asking about the characteristics of the patient's cough or headache. In addition to discussing theories of spiritual and moral development, I provided them with simple ways to ask about faith and how the patient's values might impact their medical decisions, especially in the face of serious illness or end-of-life. I can only hope as PAs in the field they are now more comfortable approaching these concerns with their patients.

Suffering

Why is there suffering? Why do good people suffer? Why does anyone have to suffer? It seems God permits suffering. Is this true? If God is creator of all, did God create suffering? If God is almighty, why doesn't God take suffering away? Suffering and sorrow are universal and bind us together as inhabitants of this imperfect world. Jack Kornfield writes in *A Path with Heart* "... in the end it is not the sorrow of the world alone that matters but our heart's response to it". So, how are we to respond to suffering?

Life with a chronic illness brings other existential questions to mind, as well. Am I still loveable even though I see myself as damaged goods? How can God still love me when I can't serve God the way I used to or would like to? How can I be useful to society in this body? How can I contribute to the betterment of the world? How do I continue a relationship with God when I'm too tired to pray?

These are heady questions with no ready answers. What is clear is that it is unlikely that a person can live a full life and escape suffering on some level. What is also clear is that we cannot fully appreciate life without death, wellness without illness, light without darkness, summer without winter, colors without black and white. Perhaps the best approach is simply acceptance of what is, of the paradoxes of life.

That said, it is difficult not to be sad about all the losses associated with living with a chronic illness, primarily about the loss of a sense of purpose to one's life. I just can't imagine God is pleased at how well I can complete a crossword puzzle or Sudoku. There must be something more to life than that. So, the chief issue now, for me, is how to find meaning in a life that seems to have no purpose.

I often remember Helen, one of the residents in a nursing home where I was chaplain. One day she asked me what I thought was her purpose in life. I turned the question back to her and after a moment she replied, "I think it's to smile and be gracious". I suspect when you get right down to it the essence of life may really be as simple as that.

I have observed many things from the perspective of a person living with a chronic illness. When someone is diagnosed with an illness, especially if it becomes chronic, and especially if the person diagnosed is young, many people react with a combination of sympathy and fear. Sympathy is easy to understand. Fear takes some exploring. Some fear stems from concerns for the welfare of the ill person. Will the person be able to continue working, earn a living, live a long life, engage in hobbies, ever be well again? Another fear is completely turned in on the self. This is the fear that drives friends, family, neighbors, coworkers away. This is the fear that if they get too close to a person who is ill, they might get sick too.

There is also the fear of facing one's own mortality. We all know we will die someday but for many that day is some nebulous date in the, hopefully, distant future. Hearing of the illness of a close friend or relative brings us front and center with the fact that this, too, could happen to me, and, in fact, will likely happen to me. One could experience a sudden and unexpected death, but generally that is not the case. Mostly our bodies gradually lose the energy, efficiency, and vigor of our younger days. One slowly experiences a decline in ability, sight, hearing, mobility, and perhaps independence. Although some go kicking and screaming the entire way to the grave, most come to a peaceful co-existence with the diminishments of old age.

But when illness comes to visit unexpectedly and arrives at your door with packed bags and an intent to take up residence in the guest room of your body, this is another situation all together. This visitor barges in, unpacks, interrupts your life, and announces, "Now, what shall we do today?" You may want to respond, "I don't know what *we* are doing but *you* are leaving". However, illness simply goes to the kitchen, makes a cup of tea, sits down opposite you and grins. Now what? That is a big question and one that cannot be answered simply, easily, or quickly.

Wishing for Death

"I wish God would stop waking me up." "I really wish I were dead." "How much longer do I have to put up with this?" "I don't want to go on living like this." "I'm so angry that I'm still here." "The only reason I'm still here is because I haven't yet found a sure way of ending my life."

I have said these words and similar ones on many occasions, sometimes only to myself but at times to others. Yet, at no time has anyone ever asked me if I had plans to kill myself, not even people with health care experience who should know that these can be warning signals. I mentioned this once to a former coworker who said that he suspected I was feeling suicidal years ago when we worked together but that he was sure I would never kill myself because I was "a good Catholic girl", as if to say Catholics never commit suicide.

The issue of death comes up frequently for me. I live in Vermont which has a death with dignity law but only those deemed to be in the last six months of life and who have been diagnosed with a terminal illness can access life-ending drugs. I struggle with this. If I make decisions or do things that others may consider foolish or stupid or unwise, but am considered legally competent, I have the right to make those decisions and do those things regardless of the opinions of others. Yet, when it comes to ending my life, I am not permitted to make that decision myself.

We will all die. Why can't a competent person make the decision to end his or her life if the person deems that life to no longer be of sufficient quality to continue living? I sincerely doubt that if we opened life-ending medications to everyone that there would be a run on them. Is it morally correct to allow people to dwindle or to force people to live lives they feel are not worth living simply so we can say we didn't put them to death? Shouldn't individuals be able to decide for themselves what constitutes a quality life?

I once asked friends to describe me in one word. The word that was used most frequently was "courageous". I don't see myself this way. Then again, perhaps I am courageous. It takes courage to continue living a life that seems pointless, and unless you live with an illness like ME you have no idea how difficult it is to carry on with no end in sight. In the late 1990's I seriously considered suicide. I saw no light at the end of the tunnel. I was unable to work more than just a few hours a week once a week and it would take my body an entire week to recover from that half shift, and then it was back to work again. My life was very limited, I was barely able to support myself financially, I saw no hope for the future being any different. I started to plan my death.

If you have never considered suicide you can't understand that when you are in that state of mind death is the most logical decision. It makes perfect sense to end your life. Why would you want to do otherwise? Why would I want to stay in a life that is meaningless, especially when, from my faith perspective, what comes after this earthly life is incredibly marvelous? It is a challenge to stay here on earth when I would rather be in heaven with God.

What a paradox this is. My faith says I should stay here because my life has value, I am a person of dignity, and there is a plan and purpose to my life. Yet my faith also seems to tell me that no matter what the circumstances I will be welcomed home by a loving and merciful God. Some would say that a person who commits suicide is condemned to eternal damnation. That's not what my God would do and that's not the kind of God I want to put my faith in. Some would call this faulty theology and perhaps it is. It is easy to twist our notions of God and of what we read in scripture to suit our own needs and desires.

So, is it a matter of faith that keeps me here? Or is it trust in God? Am I a coward not to end my life? Or have I just not yet found the best way to end my life? Or am I just masochistic? I dismiss the masochistic theory out of hand; I wish suffering as little as the next person. So, it's down to faith or trust. Or is it both? And who is this God in whom I have placed my faith and trust?

I grew up with a not-so-uncommon notion that God was the strict Father who kept a list of all the things we did right and wrong and, of course, the "wrong" list was much longer than the "right" list. Somehow, we mere mortals could just never do enough right things for God to be really pleased with us. And when we died God would look at our record and decide if we went to heaven, hell, or purgatory. Only real saints got to heaven. The rest of us were either condemned forever to hell or spent endless ages in purgatory until God felt we were perhaps now good enough to be in His presence. I learned that Jesus was this gentle being that God the Father sent to earth. Somehow his death on the cross redeemed us. The Holy Spirit was some nebulous part of the Trinity that no one talked about very much. Plus, being the "third person" of the Trinity, the Spirit was relegated to last place in the hierarchy and therefore couldn't be very important anyway. God the Father was in charge. The buck stopped with Him.

Somewhere along the line, I began to have a different understanding of God. Gradually God became more personable, more real, more like someone I could actually have a relationship with. I came to know God as compassionate, loving, caring, merciful, good, desiring to shower me with grace, desiring me to be happy and joyful, not desiring me to suffer, and waiting to welcome me home with open arms and a big hug at the end of my earthly existence. I have suffered from physical diminishment, from emotional distress, from spiritual ennui. Yet I know that God is here with me. God does not abandon God's people. This is the God who knit me together in my mother's womb and still cares for me.

This is the mystery of life. This is the question to which I have no answer other than faith and trust – that there is a purpose to every life even though that purpose may be beyond our understanding. How is God going to make sense of this life of mine? God and I chat often. I ask why I'm still here. God says wait. I ask why. God says because. I say why did I even bother asking. Not particularly insightful conversations. So, perhaps what keeps me here is curiosity.

I have no fear of death. I welcome it. When I hear others ask who would want to die, I want to wave my hands wildly in the air and say, "I do, I do". Yet I typically restrain myself. Speaking of death is not acceptable in polite company. I wonder why that is. Death will happen to all of us sooner or later. It is a given; part of being mortal.

When I die I will see God face-to-face! What a joy that will be! The anticipation of that joy is what makes it difficult to tolerate my earthly existence. It makes me want to die now. Why put it off? Why stay here when what awaits is infinitely better than anything I can experience on earth, and most especially better than the life I am experiencing in a body that functions poorly? Yet, wait I must. I'm fine with dying tomorrow but a part of me wants to live long enough for those who do not understand the challenges of a life with chronic illness to diminish to my level just so I can ask them, "Do you get it now?"

I struggle with the notion that my body is holy. I know this in my head, though getting it through to my heart is a life-long task. This overweight, flabby, chronically unwell body is holy! It was easier to think of my body as holy when it worked well. Holiness seemed akin to functionality. When I was able and strong, I felt I could serve God well.

But, I was wrong. I know that whether the body functions well or poorly has no connection to its holiness. Either way it is God's creation. God values it and it has been my job to find a way to value my body as it has diminished in its ability to function normally. This is quite a challenge especially given that I am the type of person who wants answers, who wants to know how and why. It has required me to separate my body from my being, my essence. It has required me to explore who and what I am at my core, to discover and honor the spark of the Divine that dwells in me, that has dwelt there from my conception and will until my last breath when I will be reunited fully with the Divine from Whom I came. It has required me to see a beauty in my body beyond its physical appearance.

I will be cremated when I die. The idea of cremation, of reducing the body to ashes does not sit completely comfortably with me. It seems a bit brutal, yet I know it will be painless. Cremation is customary in some cultures, necessary in others. My decision to be cremated is more of an environmental one than anything else. Why use the space in the ground as is required for a body to be buried? And why waste money and wood on an elaborate coffin that will only be relegated to the ground?

Reflecting more on the word "reduce" in connection to cremation of the body, I reflect on how my body has been reduced in its ability to function normally over the past decades. So perhaps it is appropriate that my body undergo the final reduction to ashes when my life here is finally over. Cremation can also be seen as a process of purification. Chronic illness is also a purifying and purging process. It strips a person of all the excess and leaves only what is necessary. And sometimes it leaves your life in ashes.

Several years ago, I purchased my burial urn. It seems fitting that after death my human remains will dwell in a beautiful container. I entered the world from a beautiful and small container and will leave the world in a beautiful and small container. My urn sits atop the armoire in my bedroom. With myalgic encephalomyelitis, I spend more time in bed than do most people, sometimes sleeping, sometimes just resting. But as I look around the room my eyes fall on my urn, my final earthly resting place. I enjoy looking at my urn. I enjoy the comfort of knowing where my bodily remains will dwell after I die. I am pleased that it stands ready to receive me.

I chose this particular urn because it reflects my love of nature. The design is simple – white with a painted hummingbird on the wing – and for the present serves as a thing of beauty in my home. It seems an appropriate final resting place for me, a simple container for a person who tries to live a simple life.

Is it a bit odd to have spent time searching for the perfect urn, one that reflects who I am, what I value, that says something about me? After all, once I am dead the urn will be unimportant to me. So, is the appearance of the urn more for me or for my survivors? Perhaps it's both. It comforts me now and I hope it will comfort my survivors to carry me to my grave in something that reflects the beauty of nature. Perhaps they will recall times spent on my porch watching the hummingbirds flit from feeder to feeder and chatter away as they protect their territory. The hummers don't stay here year-round so perhaps the hummingbird on the urn will remind my survivors that we all have to migrate to new places in life and someday embark on our final migration at death.

Struggles and Attitudes

Commonly, there is little recognition of the struggles those with chronic illnesses encounter daily. For me it may be because to a certain extent I hid the depth my symptoms. I felt I needed to keep up the appearance of wellness in family relationships and with employers and coworkers as well. If my employers knew how poorly I felt and how much I struggled to think, process, show up at work, and be cheerful when I felt miserable, I'm sure I would have lost my job. Eventually, I did.

My life with chronic illness is often accompanied by bitterness and anger. A portion of those feelings are directed toward the health care system that has been unable to find out what's wrong with my body and affect a cure. I say this knowing full well that, as I discussed previously, we know very little about how the body works and especially about the connections between mind, body, and spirit.

The bitterness also stems from a lack of compassion towards me and, by extension, all those who are chronically ill. I realize it's impossible for those who have relatively healthy bodies or who are experiencing the normal aches and pains and diminishments of aging to understand what life is like for those who have been living with chronic illness for most of their lives but often there is little effort to understand.

Bitterness and anger also stem from having been deprived, in the prime of my life, of the life I expected and hoped to live. All my energy went into earning a living and maintaining my independence. There was no energy left for fun.

I don't want pity. Pity seems to have an air of contempt; feeling sorry for someone from the perspective that if the person was just stronger or had more gumption that person would just get over whatever it is that has a hold on the person and get on with life. I want to be treated with compassion. Compassion accompanies a person with a desire to spare the person from suffering. It is a willingness to be with the suffering person, not as one who understands (for who can truly understand what another is experiencing) but simply as a companion, as one who cares.

People seem to find it easy to be compassionate toward someone who is ill or suffering if that situation has a clear ending. We can feel for and do our best to assist a person who has the flu or a hip replacement, knowing that our services – be that chicken soup or a trip to physical therapy – are temporary. But if the situation is chronic then compassion fatigue sets in. That leaves those with chronic illness at the whim of others' time and kindness.

When I was teaching at a physician assistant program the program director was aware that my health was less than stellar, yet one day when I came to work feeling very tired but ready to teach my class she declared "your illness is not my problem". As true as that statement was (after all, she was not responsible for my being ill) her statement seemed to lack any understanding, compassion, or willingness to hear how difficult it was for a person to work with less than a full tank of energy. Somehow, I was expected to leave my fatigue at home. Then again, my illness in some way *was* her problem in that if one of us is hurting we are all hurting. If one of us is sick, we are all sick. And until all of us are well, none of us is completely well.

I found a similar attitude when working in a parish setting. When the pastor hired me I was honest with him about my chronic condition yet somehow I was also expected not to be ill or at least not to have illness ever interfere with my work.

At a nursing home where I was employed as a chaplain, I was labeled as "unreliable" because my symptoms flared on the day a special event was scheduled and I was unable to work. I had a small role assigned to me for that event that was easily covered by another staff member, yet I was "unreliable" from that day onward.

Am I unreliable? Now I am, for sure. One of the hallmarks of this mystery illness is "non-restorative sleep" which means that no matter how much sleep I get I never feel refreshed. It's as if I haven't slept at all. I feel as tired (and as grumpy) when I awaken as I did when I went to bed. Additionally, I have the typical "brain fog" that sometimes makes simple tasks such as driving ten minutes down familiar roads into an experience akin to driving with sunglasses on at night and in reverse gear. So, yes, I sometimes cancel appointments at the last minute because I need to go back to bed. And, yes, I cancel a lunch date at the last minute because I realized as I was leaving the driveway that I wasn't able to attend to all the sensory input driving requires and my reaction time was nil. Unreliable, yes. Intentionally, no.

Perhaps it has to do with our attitude in this culture toward those who are in less than perfect health. It's as if we are contagious – stay away, it might be catching. The unhealthy are looked upon as stupid – how could you let this happen to yourself – the same way we may look at obese people, like me now, and wonder how they could let themselves become so fat. Clearly these happen because the person is lazy.

Our culture equates what you do for work with who you are. Productive people are valued. If you are not working or are on disability or receive public assistance or food stamps it must be because you are lazy. That seems to be the default reaction when in reality there are many reasons why a person may not be able to secure, or keep, gainful employment or have enough money to pay the bills.

In the midst of not working, it is difficult to maintain a sense of dignity and a sense of identity. I suspect everyone wants to work, to be useful, to contribute to the betterment of society. This makes us feel good about ourselves. Working gives us the opportunity to support ourselves, to provide for our needs and the needs of those dependent on us. When work is taken away, especially when that taking away is out of one's control, it takes a toll on one's self-image.

We who carry chronic illness with us as others carry their American Express card (we don't leave home without it!) are not this way intentionally. We simply want to be loved, despite of our frailties. We want to be treated with dignity. Underneath the fatigue, the occasional irritability because we're running on empty all the time, the need to take extra time to rest, the need to reduce sensory stimulation, is a desire to be respected for our abilities, not denigrated for our disabilities.

What I have experienced as a lack of compassion from various people in a variety of settings I could also term abandonment. Others might call it cruelty, meanness, or intolerance and certainly there is an element of all of these. I suspect that anyone who has a chronic illness that interferes with the ordinary tasks of life has also experienced abandonment. I have been abandoned and have abandoned others. It's a simple fact that some people don't have the time or desire to befriend a person who cannot hold up the other end of the friendship. Likely they would have abandoned me anyway, perhaps when I moved or disagreed with them on a topic dear to their heart. Some I suspect leave the relationship out of fear. It can be scary to be around someone who is not well. It is a reminder that sooner or later their body will fail, too. Others tire of being stood-up and misinterpret cancellation of plans as an indication that I no longer want their friendship when the truth is that I cannot function on that particular day.

I have abandoned people who have high energy levels and those who are what I would term "high maintenance". The truth is that I just can't tolerate what I refer to as "sensory overload" – lots of movement, noise, talking, certain decibel levels, being in a crowd, and I don't have the energy to give to people who need constant validation or attention. It may be cruel but sooner or later it comes to a matter of self-preservation. So, a person learns who is healthy to be around and who is not. The difficulty for relationships is that all this can change from day to day or even from hour to hour. It is difficult enough for the ill person to adjust to these vagaries; asking others to do so is sometimes beyond their capabilities. I realize that just as sometimes I simply can't have a certain person in my life, the shoe also fits on the other foot. I can be too heavy a load for others to handle.

Those who have stayed with me through the years are precious people capable of seeing beyond the illness to the person underneath. Perhaps they see with the eyes of God.

You Just Don't Get It

As I've said, it is difficult, if not impossible, for those who are well to understand the world of those who are ill. I sat across from a friend of over thirty years at our favorite restaurant one day and used every power within me not to look her straight in the eyes and say "F*** you". She was trying to convince me that I would benefit from a treatment I felt was completely inappropriate. To her, and others full of suggestions, I simply want to say, "you just don't get it".

You just don't get it that there's a difference between sadness and depression although the words are often used interchangeably. Clinical depression seems to be caused by a problem with neurotransmitters in the brain. Sadness or sorrow is caused by life events.

You just don't get it that my desire for solitude and quiet is not simply anti-social behavior. Sensory input of just about any kind can overwhelm me. Too many people in a room, crisscrossing conversations, loud voices, children's voices and their energy level, music, and stimulating visual input are just too much to bear. So, no, I'm not interested in going to the community potluck. I'm not interested in spending time with you when your grandchildren are visiting. I'm not interested in going to a concert. I won't be attending the family reunion. Please can we sit in a quiet corner of the restaurant or let's meet at my house for a quiet meal instead. It's not that I don't want to be sociable, it's simply that I have to limit my sensory exposure as a matter of self-preservation.

You just don't get it that my excess weight is not from overeating. In reality, I have little appetite. But my life is sedentary and that does not help a body stay slim. My body just doesn't seem to work well and part of that not working well is not processing food properly.

You just don't get it that I'm not interested in trying some treatment you heard about or saw on the internet. Over the 30+ years I've been dealing with this mystery illness I've tried just about everything – antibiotics (both oral and intravenous), traditional Chinese medicine, homeopathy, naturopathy, acupuncture and acupressure, Reiki, and any number of supplements and vitamin combinations. I've tried dairy-free, gluten-free, caffeine-free, sugar-free. I've had blood tests, and scans, and neurological testing, and been poked and prodded and yet no definitive diagnosis has been forthcoming. I've seen family doctors, internists, infectious disease specialists, neurologists, psychologists, orthopedists, rheumatologists, and hematologists. No treatment has worked and I do not have the emotional reserve to be disappointed once again. If that sounds defeatist to you, then so be it.

You just don't get it that I need to live here in Vermont. It is a place of safety and security for me. Here I'm nourished by the beauty of the landscape, and, yes, by the snow that falls in abundance each winter. That's not to say that I appreciate day upon day of high temperatures below zero but that's just part of winter in the North Country. Summer makes up for that, even in its brevity. Here I am loved and cared for. Here I can find that a box of blueberries has mysteriously found its way to my porch, or perhaps some fresh flowers. Here a gallon of milk will appear if I can't get out to the store. Yes, these things can happen in other places but it's a certainty here.

You just don't get it that life with chronic illness is reduced to the necessities of life with little room left for pithy things like whether or not your lawn mower needs repair or your grandchild will need braces. It's not that I don't care, it's that I don't have the energy to care. As a consequence of chronic illness my world has become very small. My energy is used to take a shower, get to the store, make a simple meal. Not much is left over for other concerns. What matters is how I will get through today.

You just don't get it that even though I look like an overweight but otherwise healthy person I am not. So when I leave the post office because I can't stand that long in line it's not because I expect instant service, it's because when I stand for any period of time I feel weak and in need of a chair post-haste. When you see me pull into a handicap parking spot it's not that I'm lazy, it's that I have a thimble-full of energy and I choose not to use it walking extra steps to my destination. And when I say that I'm on disability, it's not because I'm gaming the system, it's because I truly am unable to hold down a job.

Life with chronic illness is not for the faint of heart. It is not something anyone wishes for. It is something that knocks unexpectedly on the door, comes in, unpacks its bags, and settles in for the long run. So, what's a person to do? Pick a fight or put on the tea kettle and settle in for a chat?

Please! No Platitudes!

It is difficult to know what to say to someone who never feels well. Here are some common statements that are not helpful.

"I know how you feel." Well, unless you also have a chronic illness that takes your energy away and leaves your life in a shambles, you don't know how I feel. Please do not pretend you do.

"God has a plan for you." Really? You can read God's mind? Amazing! According to my theology God's plan is for us to love one another. My God does not have a planning calendar for each individual person. I don't think even God could keep track of us all, given how our freedom to choose can intentionally or unintentionally interfere with someone else's life.

"Tomorrow will be a better day." How do you know? Do you have a crystal ball that reads the future? Tomorrow may actually be worse than today so please don't promise me something you can't. The sun may not come out tomorrow.

"Everything happens for a reason." Do you really believe that? The tornado that killed so many? The flood that took out the motor home park? The mass shooting that took innocent lives? I'm not saying that good things cannot come out of bad but to make a blanket statement that there is a reason, as if pre-ordained, for every life event seems a bit Pollyanna-ish.

"Just take it one day at a time." Well, how else am I supposed to take my life? Two days at a time? A week at a time? Sometimes I need to take life one hour at a time. With this illness it is impossible to look too far into the future since symptoms can change from morning to afternoon to evening. I have to take life as it presents itself.

"Have you tried (fill in the blank with a treatment you've heard of but may never have tried)." Trust me. I've tried everything within reason and a few options on the margins. I am done with that. I cannot get my hopes up once again and risk having them dashed. If someone had a definitive treatment I'd take it. Otherwise, it seems better to just cope with what I have.

"Look what so-and-so did with his/her/their life." I am only me. I can only do what works for me. I can only respond to an illness from my perspective and according to my personality and strengths and weaknesses. Yes, I can learn from how others have dealt with adversity but in the end I can only be me.

◌

I know you are just trying to help and be kind but, please, no platitudes. Spend a day or a week in my body and then see what you'd like people to say to you. Perhaps something like this:

"I cannot imagine how you feel."

"I don't know if I could tolerate what you put up with all the time."

"I'm sorry this is happening to you."

"I wish I could take all this away."

"You don't deserve this."

"I don't know what to say."

"I wish I had the words/means to help you feel better."

"What would be most helpful for you today?"

"I love you and I care."

Now

The question "How are you?" seems simple but is actually quite complex. When asked this question my response depends on the situation and the person asking. If it's a casual contact on the street or in the grocery store my response typically is the usual "Fine. How are you?". But if the question is asked by someone who really wants to know then I may respond "Do you want the socially acceptable answer or the truth?" And what is the truth?

The truth is that I'm tired. I'm spent. I'm exhausted. And I'm tired of being tired, spent, and exhausted.

I am living in a type of limbo between life and death. When I was young and attending Catholic grade school the nuns told us that limbo was the place where unbaptized babies went or where you went as a punishment if you didn't go straight to heaven or straight to hell. It was a sort of waiting room for heaven, like purgatory. Only saints went straight to heaven. And if you were bound for hell, you went straight there.

But I have discovered that limbo is here on earth, that place where you wait either for something better here or you wait for death. And since living with a chronic illness such as ME is sufficient punishment, I'm on the express train to heaven!

If I could have some sense of purpose to my life perhaps that sense of living in limbo would ease. I became symptomatic in 1987 and my body finally protested too much to continue working in 2013 at age 58. Given that ME is not a fatal illness and I am now already ten years older than I was when I stopped working and I'm still here, the question of the purpose of my life is quite prominent.

I know I need to extend compassion towards myself. This is difficult because I've been putting out the image of a capable woman for so many years – or at least I hope so! Some of the difficulty comes from my upbringing where what was modeled for me was being stoic, not complaining, suffering in silence, offering up difficulties for the souls in purgatory, and not being a burden. And I've been afraid of being seen as a failure – something I always felt I was as I was growing up because I saw myself as not as intelligent as my siblings. I was the dumb one. I had to show them and myself that I could make it on my own.

These days I need to be gentle with and kind toward myself and take extraordinarily good care of myself in the small ways I am still able to do. I also need to forgive myself. Even though I'm not sure as I review my life that I would change past decisions there is on some level a sense that I brought this illness on myself, all the while knowing that is not true. Life happens quickly and although I do feel I made the decisions that were right at the time perhaps they were not right for the long run.

Adopting gratitude is helpful. I am grateful for the independence, self-sufficiency, and solitude I have; a warm and safe place to live, good friends nearby, caring family, functioning car with gas in the tank, money to pay the bills, food at the ready, clothes to wear, a comfortable bed, quiet surroundings. I am grateful for time to contemplate, to watch the snow fall, to watch the clouds go by, observe the antics of the hummingbirds and listen to the ratchety call of the orioles, and to have few demands on my time.

I also appreciate the unexpected benefits of illness. I can do with less money because I am unable to travel and have few needs. I can do with less "stuff". I know who my real friends are. I have learned to say no. I have learned to accept help from others. I continue to learn that I am more than what I do. I am more gentle with myself. I have given myself permission to do less. I continue to shed useless things. I have learned to ask for help and not put all the pressure on myself to do everything for fear of appearing weak or stupid. I have learned to trust that God will provide for what I truly need. I have more compassion towards those who are ill. I am slowly learning to reverence myself.

Yet, I must confess, I covet. I covet many things. Primarily I covet those people blessed with energy, people who can plan their day/week/year and proceed through it with an air of certainty that their body will cooperate with those plans. I used to have that body. It's almost like a dream now it's been so long. I've become accustomed to all my plans being tentative. I covet more certainty. I covet the ability to make commitments and be reasonably sure I can keep them.

I feel for my family and friends. They mean well and wish to help but there is little they can do. I suspect they sometimes feel helpless, and I feel helpless to help them. They can't affect a cure. They can't wave a magic wand over me and make me well again. There is little I need in the way of material assistance. I hope they believe that I'm doing my best and that they can continue to simply be there for me.

And I am doing my best. I'm coping in the only way I know how. I'm not doing what others do or feeling what others feel or taking the steps others take because I'm not those others. I am me and can only do what works for me.

I have been given the gift of time. Many people don't receive this. They die young or drop dead at work and never have the time to simply rest. I don't ever have to hurry, which is a good thing because I don't do it well! I have what many people crave — the time to enjoy the scenery, watch a winter storm come in, look for the rainbow after a summer thunderstorm, read to my heart's content, nap whenever I want. I have not been very good at waiting for whatever is next, be that tomorrow, next year, or ten years from now. Because my life is not as I wish it to be, I tend to focus too far into the future, to death and the life to come. I will always yearn to see God face to face but am trying to focus more on the grace that is always there to help me live in the present.

So, for now, I get up and go through the day, doing what needs to be done, wandering to the mailbox and, when necessary, beyond, and finish out the day. The next day I get up....

Final Thoughts

A few final words. I hope this book has accomplished its aim of educating and providing some insight into a life with Myalgic Encephalomyelitis. Perhaps it even brought comfort in knowing you are not alone if you, too, live with ME.

Because there is no known cause for ME, treatment is problematic. There is no magic pill to make the symptoms go away and for life to return to normal.

That said, here are some things that may help:

Most importantly, be kind to yourself. You didn't cause this to happen. It's not your fault. It's not because of anything you did or didn't do. It's most likely because something got triggered in your immune system, probably from some viral illness, and whatever switch got turned on or off never got flipped back the other way.

Accept your situation. You have ME and it's unlikely to go away, so you need to find some way to make peace with it. You may be able to do this yourself, particularly if your symptoms are not too debilitating. You may need to seek professional help from a psychologist or counselor. Try to find one who is interested in and has experience with chronic illness. It is a unique experience and many of the approaches that work for other illnesses or life experiences just don't apply to learning to live with ME. Perhaps a support group in your area or one you can connect to online would be helpful. No one can help you cope with ME or understand what you are experiencing better than someone in the same shoes.

Learn to live within your limits. We all need to do this whether we are well or ill. People with a chronic illness need to be that much more attentive to their limits. This may seem restrictive but in the long run it is to your benefit and the benefit of those you love and who love you and care about you.

Rest. This is vital. Your body heals with rest and sleep so do as much of either or both as you need. This may mean you have to rearrange your life but that's part of learning to live with ME. Rest in as quiet and as comfortable a place as you can.

Take stock of what is most important in your life and put your energy there. Let everything else go. Sometimes this means letting go of relationships as well. Things/events/people that sap your energy are not helpful. You may not be able to drop them or change their influence on your life immediately but consider making what changes you can as soon as you can.

Elicit the help of family or friends, neighbors or acquaintances, or local agencies who may be able to help you with what needs to be done that you can no longer do yourself, or that you just don't have the energy at the moment to do. Many people, myself included, have difficulty asking for help. We feel weak or as if we have failed in some way. And then there is the fear of losing our independence. Put those feelings aside for the time being and ask for help remembering that just because you need help today doesn't mean you will always need it.

Many people will be certain they know what is best for you. They may indeed have good ideas that you should consider incorporating into your life, but you are the best to decide what you need and what you don't. Feel free to say "no", or "not right now", or "thank you for the offer; perhaps some other time".

Try not to over-extend yourself. It is impossible to predict how you will feel from day to day, or even from morning to afternoon to evening, so if the option is to do more or to do less, choose less. You can always do more later. The world will not end if the dishes sit in the sink for another day. Perhaps several smaller trips to the grocery store would be better for your energy level than one big food shopping expedition.

Be kind to your brain. If you find you can't read, then don't. If you need to write things down in order to remember them, then do so. Do whatever your brain is capable of and no more.

Reputable ME websites or the CDC offer other tips for coping with ME and how to talk with your health care provider and your family and friends about your new life. Consider taking advantage of what they have to offer.

All the best to you!

Recommended Reading

Doka, Kenneth J., Ed. *Living with Grief When Illness is Prolonged.* London and New York: Routledge, 2016.

Duff, Kat. *The Alchemy of Illness.* New York: Bell Tower, 1993.

Earle, Mary C. *Broken Body, Healing Spirit.* Harrisburg, PA: Morehouse Publishing, 2003.

Earle, Mary C. *Beginning Again.* Harrisburg, PA: Morehouse Publishing, 2004.

Elliot, Elisabeth. *A Path Through Suffering: Discovering the Relationship Between God's Mercy and Our Pain.* Ann Arbor, MI: Servant Publications, 1990.

Gawande, Atul. *Being Mortal.* New York: Picador Publishing, 2017.

Kornfield, Jack. *A Path with Heart.* New York: Random House, 1993.

Kubler-Ross, Elisabeth, MD. *On Death and Dying.* New York: Scribner, 1997.

Pert, Candace, PhD. *The Molecules of Emotion.* New York: Scribner, 1999.

Rehm, Diane. *When My Time Comes.* New York: Knopf-Doubleday Publishing Group, 2021.

Rohr, Richard, OFM. *Things Hidden.* Cincinnati, OH: Franciscan Media, 2008.

Ross, Susan. *Chronic Sorrow.* London and New York: Routledge, 2002.

Acknowledgements

Gratitude and thanks go to my insightful readers: Tom Baker, Amy Borgman, Pam Hanson, Sandy Lucas, and Diane Williams. Your comments, honesty, and encouragement were vital to the completion of this project. Special thanks to Pam for her slide puzzle reworking of one chapter, and to Tom for transforming the manuscript into book form.

Many thanks to Deb Schonberg for graciously contributing her talents for the cover illustration.

❧

The author invites your comments at
www.beyondthemailbox.net.